MY CHOICE, MY DESTINY

T0158945

My Choice, My Destiny

My Kidney Transplant Journey

Mina Gonzales

iUniverse LLC
Bloomington

My Choice, My Destiny
My Kidney Transplant Journey

iUniverse books may be ordered through booksellers or by contacting:

iUniverse LLC
1663 Liberty Drive
Bloomington, IN 47403
www.iuniverse.com
1-800-Authors (1-800-288-4677)

Because of the dynamic nature of the Internet, any web addresses or links contained in this book may have changed since publication and may no longer be valid. The views expressed in this work are solely those of the author and do not necessarily reflect the views of the publisher, and the publisher hereby disclaims any responsibility for them.

Any people depicted in stock imagery provided by Thinkstock are models, and such images are being used for illustrative purposes only.
Certain stock imagery © Thinkstock.

ISBN: 978-1-4917-0337-3 (sc)
ISBN: 978-1-4917-0339-7 (hc)
ISBN: 978-1-4917-0338-0 (ebk)

Library of Congress Control Number: 2013915170

Printed in the United States of America

iUniverse rev. date: 08/24/2013

CONTENTS

This book is dedicated to all the kidney transplant patients who come after me. I hope they find solace in my story of kidney transplantation and that they find their rainbow at the end of dialysis and an angel of their own.

FOREWORD

Dedication, determination and a desire to do good by others is the passion that drives Mina Gonzales. Her goal is to provide a guideline for others who suffer or will suffer the same plight as she; kidney failure and finally transplantation.

Mina presents a no holds barred honest approach to sharing her story, her journey from near death to fifteen years as a kidney transplant survivor. Although vulnerable to possible personal retribution, she tells it like it is.

In her book, "My Choice, My Destiny: My Kidney Transplant Journey", Mina shares the not so good days with a fresh outlook to the possible consequences that come with kidney failure. And she shares the good days with a renewed joy and love of life. She presents a bold and determined mental and spiritual understanding of what really was happening, what her options were, possible outcomes and her final victory; a successful kidney transplant.

I encourage all who read this book, whether because you find yourself facing the same heart wrenching life threatening kidney disease, or because you know someone, a family member or close friend who is similarly suffering, that you share this book with them. I guarantee they will gain insight, recognize some of what they are going through and hopefully find solace in knowing that a healthy long life can be had after kidney transplantation and that there is always hope. That is what Mina found out and why she chose to share "My Choice, My Destiny: My Kidney Transplant Journey" with you.

Denise L. Cook, Editor/Writer

ORACLE Publishing

PREFACE

Life is a journey, and I believe we are all put on this earth for a purpose.

—Mina Gonzales

I did a lot of soul searching. I feel my breath rising and falling inside my chest, and I can feel my heartbeat. I am new again. I am no longer just walking through my life on autopilot—I am moving with life. I am not the stupid person I believed myself to be.

My mission in life is not merely to survive, but to thrive and to do so with some passion, some compassion, some humor, and some style.

—Maya Angelou

Every day may not be perfect, but I thank God for each day of my life.

> Sometimes, the paths that we take are long and hard,
> but those are the ones with the most beautiful views.
>
> —Collin McCarty

It took me several years to realize that as long as we do not listen to people who try to project their own insecurities on us, we have the opportunity to accomplish our dreams and goals every day. Life is too short and precious.

I am a pioneer. When I face a new challenge, I try to take my beginning wherever it may be and start from there. I have overcome lots of obstacles in my life, but I learned that I have to control my fears or my fears will control me. Dialysis was one of the obstacles to overcome. I don't think I could have gone through it without the love of my family. We must take the opportunity every day to live life to the fullest.

> A journey of a thousand miles begins with a single step.
>
> —Laozi

You can see the scars of dialysis, but you cannot see the scars of the heart and soul. There is negative and positive in everybody's life. Know that the positive will always propel you forward. The negative allows you to learn from your mistakes and become a better person. This is how I learned that I deserved to live without other people setting me back. This was my choice and my destiny!

ACKNOWLEDGMENTS

I couldn't decide how best to say thank you to those who helped me along on journey from illness. The best way I knew how was to tell each of their stories.

I want to thank my angel who saved my life, my organ donor, and his family. In spite of their grief, these people thought of others. My husband dedicated seven years of his life to take care of me. My grandson was my inspiration to keep fighting.

These special people also shared my journey.

Brenda Chemleski: Brenda was a nurse (RN/CNN) who worked at Kaiser. She has held many positions during her career, all in the renal field. She is now retired. Brenda deserves to have a whole book about her and all the wonderful things she has done, but I'm going to sum up how amazing she was to me. I met Brenda at Kaiser in Los Angeles, California, on the worst day of my life. I had just found out that hemodialysis wasn't working for me anymore. If I couldn't get a transplant, I would die. I then heard of another type of dialysis called peritoneal dialysis. It was only an experimental procedure. This wonderful lady with a big smile on her face entered my hospital room and said, "Hi, my name is Brenda, and I'm going to teach you about peritoneal dialysis."

I looked at her and rudely said, "Get out of my room. I'm not going to do peritoneal!" She looked back at me with such compassion and told me to call her whenever I was ready. After a couple of days, I called her, but only because it was my only choice. She then scheduled me for an emergency surgery, and the training took place a few days later.

To this day, I see Brenda as my mentor because she taught me the meaning of compassion and self-awareness for others. A few years after my transplant, I got a job as an educator working at different dialysis centers. It didn't matter if I was having troubles at home—as soon as I walked into the dialysis center, I had a smile on my face because I remembered my mentor. I was taught to educate the patients from a manual, but because of Brenda, I learned to work from the heart with the patients. Brenda, thank you for everything you have done for me. Don't stop being the amazing person you are.

Olga Botello: One day, I was talking to Olga about my manuscript and how I wanted to turn it into a book. She said she would put the manuscript into a book form for me. I thanked her with the thought of it not actually happening, because I had just met Olga. While on dialysis three times a week, she still found the time and patience to put together the manuscript, all while putting up with my indecisiveness. There are no words to thank her for organizing my manuscript, because she actually followed through with what she promised.

Lillian Marmol: I would also like to acknowledge Lily. She was an RN at the Glendora Artificial Kidney center. After dialyzing for three months in Los Angeles, I was transferred there. She took the time to talk to me and calm my fears. She was always there for me and the other patients, always putting us at ease with her jokes and perky personality. When I started having problems with my graft, she was always there to comfort me. As much as I hated being there, Lily always made it a positive experience. I even named my dialysis machine after her. Thank you so much, Lily, for helping me through a difficult time in my life.

Carolina Meyers: I met Carol more than twenty years ago. She was a volunteer coordinator for the National Kidney Foundation. Carol and

I worked together in numerous events sponsored by the National Kidney Foundation. We had lost touch, but started communicating again a few years ago. Even though we had lost track of each other, she still knew of me because coverage of me in the media. No matter how busy she was, she was always there for me through the good and the bad. I would like to thank her for financially helping me with making my dream of publishing my book come true.

Jean Bonnette: Jean is a social worker at Kaiser. She went above and beyond her job description with me.

Laura Guzman: Thank you for all the hours you spent transferring my book files from CD to paper. You made the book writing and publishing process easier, and I appreciate all that you did to help make my dream of publishing this book a reality.

Dora Calderon: Dora and I have been friends for four or five years. We have shared laughter and tears. Dora has been there for me through good times and bad times, whether for transportation or while working on my book. I helped her out of depression, a side effect of taking antirejection medicine. I think we helped each other. I will always be grateful for her friendship, and I know we will always continue to be friends. We will always share the fact that we each share another life inside us through our angel donors.

Denise L. Cook: Last but not least, I would like to acknowledge Denise L. Cook, my editor at Oracle and friend. Thank you for all your patience and understanding. I will always be grateful.

There were so many who were there for me. Thank you all so much. I wish I could mention you all. Please know that I appreciate you and thank you for helping me through some of the most life changing events in my life.

Chapter 1

You Can Pick Your Friends, but Not Your Family

My life is wonderful today. I live one day at a time. I wake up every morning and thank God for giving me the sunrise. Before I go to bed, I thank Him for the sunset. I get up daily free of pain and free of trying to please others. I have a relationship with God and a loving relationship with my family. Every day, I pray for God to give me the strength to carry out my mission of educating the public about organ donation.

My story does not begin so simply. Let me walk you through my journey. I was born in 1952 in Mexico. By 1955, at the age of three, my parents, two sisters, and I immigrated to the United States and made our home in Azusa, California. When I was five, I had a stroke caused by an aneurysm, which affected my left side. As children do, I adapted and adjusted.

Even though my father had a limited education, he was from a white-collar family of lawyers, doctors, and bankers. My mother came from a background of poverty. She was very insecure about herself and raised me in that fashion. She projected her own insecurities onto me. Everything was about her. Because of this experience, I no longer listen to negative people.

My parents were very hardworking people. In fact, they were always working and didn't always show their love for us. Reflecting on those days, I think that it was that they didn't know how to express their feelings. Sometimes, I felt like I received more love from my babysitter.

I remember receiving love and affection from my babysitter during the week. I was spoon-fed by my nanny, Sessy, who was a sixty-five-year-old lady and was like a grandma to me. On the weekends, though, our family spent time together. During this time, we would go to the park and when I was younger our family travelled abroad, by all appearances, we were a regular family. In public, I was my mom's little princess. I had the best clothes, we traveled, and everything appeared perfect. But it was all fake.

I know my parents made mistakes, just like I made mistakes raising my kids. At times, my mom was very abusive, but I have made peace with that and forgiven her. When you hold on to resentments the only person you hurt is yourself!

In spite of it all, I think I lived a pretty normal childhood, even through my teenage years. My life was pretty normal, whatever normal is. When you come from a dysfunctional family, normal is just what your life is. I grew up early, having to translate Spanish to English by the time I was ten. Your experience is your only reference. I grew up this way. This is the reason I am so loving with my grandkids and family, showing love now rather than later. I believe that when you are in the right place at the right time, lessons are there to be learned. I would never change anything that happened because it all made me the person I am today. This poem is how I felt at times and how I got through it:

i need to breathe

i need to breathe

to keep from killing my Spirit

i need to breathe

to keep my Faith, my Sanity, my Consciousness

i need to breathe

i need to breathe the Word

to keep peace with G-D

i need to breathe

to cleanse the heart of the Universe

i need to breathe

so what's stopping You?

just Breathe

—Denise L. Cook

I went to Azusa High School and had a lot of friends. I never liked school. To me, high school was a place where I could put my books down and take off with friends for the day. At the time, it was easy for me to blame my mom for my not liking school. It's easy when you grow up in an abusive home not to accept some responsibility and to blame others, but that's not the way life really is. In reality, you have to accept responsibility for your actions. As a teenager, I was at the stage where I rebelled against the world as it was.

I went from one party to another, from one place to another. My mother never found out what I was doing—or so I thought. To me, it was challenge, like a joke. I don't know if she knew, but if she did know, she didn't *really* know what was going on. I graduated in 1971.

CHAPTER 2

My Knight in Shining Armor

Don't Leave Go of My Hands

Don't leave go of my hands, Lord

For you are my guiding light

Don't leave go of my hands, Lord

For you guide me both day and night

Don't leave go of my hands, Lord

For I dare not be alone

Don't leave go of my hands, Lord

Please stay in my Heart, your Home

—A prayer from the Oracle

I met my husband-to-be, Richard, in June 1975. I was twenty-two at the time, and I was on cloud nine. I had finally met someone who would truly respect me. I would be loved as I had never been loved before, and he would be kind.

Six months later, on December 20, 1975, we got married. We married very young, and I thought he was my prince. My knight in shining armor was going to swoop me on to his white horse. We would ride off into the sunset, away from the problems I was having at home. In my imagination, he was going to be the one who was going to save me. I was so relieved to get on his white horse! I was the princess who believed in fairy tales! However, that wasn't the way it was. Reality hit me within a few months, and the roller coaster started from that point on. I met my husband with the hopes that he was going to save me from drowning, but my husband came with his own set of dysfunctional baggage. It was utter chaos in our home. We were both so young and immature, and we had a rocky start to our marriage. What I didn't realize was that I was the one who had growing up to do. I was the one who had to stop living in fantasyland and grow up. It seemed like I was blaming others for my unhappiness my whole life, but I discovered what was missing in my life: I had to learn to love myself.

A year later, the joy in my life came. I had my first son, Richard, my precious little baby with big green eyes. I was so filled with love when I held that little baby in my arms. I loved him so much. In February 1978, God gave me another little angel, my second son, Carlos.

It was hard raising kids. At times, it felt like I was raising those kids by myself. I was having issues in my marriage, so my entire focus was on my children. I was busy going to PTA meetings and being the football team mom. It seemed that the years passed by quickly, and I was living life on life's terms.

I didn't have a handbook, and I made a lot of mistakes raising my children. I hope they can forgive me for the mistakes I made. I have made amends to my sons. Every parent wants to do better than their own parents did. I learned to turn things around and be a better mother. I can only hope that they remember the kind of person that I am today. I am someone who has always been there for them, through good and bad times, teaching them not just by words, but by my example, and I am someone who taught them to never give up on their dreams. I want them to know that I am only a phone call away. They know that they are my world, and I always will be available for my children.

My youngest son was often ill, and he became very asthmatic by the time he was three. He was in and out of the hospital, and I thought he would die more than once. I went from one doctor to another, from one specialist to another, and my son just seemed to get worse. Whenever my son was having an asthma attack, I would tell him a special story. I would spend all night with him in my arms. I would tell him a story of the blue Smurfs. My son still remembers the story.

Time passed so quickly. Before I knew it, I was dealing with dialysis and two teenage boys. My son's asthma was still an issue, and they were both having trouble in school. I had to meet with teachers, counselors, and even the principal. I was always double parked. I didn't know whether I was coming or going. It seemed I never had time for myself

I started dialysis when my older son was seventeen. At the same time, I was also taking care of my mother, who was in her eighties and had Parkinson's disease. My dad had died, so my mother came to live with us. We all helped in her care, my sons, my husband, and I. Without a doubt, my family was my saving grace because I could not have cared for her without them. I didn't drive, so my husband drove her back and forth to the doctor appointments, but I was the translator. Needless to say, my translating skills from childhood had been perfected by this time. When I think back on those days, now that my two boys are grown and out of the house, I realize life is such an amazing gift!

Chapter 3

The Day My Life Changed

Life is never what you expect it to be, and I never thought I was headed for such a dramatic turn of events. My doctors told me that I had been fighting high blood pressure that in turn had caused my kidneys to slowly deteriorate over the course of ten years. After the tenth year I had began feeling sick. I started to feel dizzy and like I was going to pass out and figured I just didn't feel good. Days, months, and even years passed by, and every once in a while, I would feel sick. I was always tired. One day I got out of bed and just collapsed. I couldn't take another step. My blood pressure had skyrocketed to 210/110, nearly twice what it should be. High blood pressure is known as the silent killer because it often doesn't produce any signs or symptoms to warn you that you have a problem. You can have high blood pressure for years without ever knowing it. In fact, according to a Kaiser patient pamphlet, about fifteen million Americans have no idea their blood pressure is too high.

After I collapsed, my husband rushed me to a clinic. I needed more tests, so they sent me to Kaiser Sunset in Los Angeles. Once there, they wanted to admit me. I was told I had water in my lungs and possibly a kidney infection. I was told I would probably be in the hospital for just a couple of days and that they were going to perform some tests to find out what was wrong. In the meantime, they needed to control my high blood pressure.

A couple of days in the hospital turned into almost a month and a half. They did all the tests they needed to do. One day, as I was watching television, a group of specialists in stiff white coats came shuffling into my room. They turned the television off and said, "Mrs. Gonzales, you are going to die." Panic took over my whole being, and I was paralyzed with fear—all I knew was that I was going to die! The doctor told me I had three months to live, and I passed out.

While I was passed out, I had a beautiful dream that I was in heaven and that everything was luscious and green. There were flowers, trees, and rivers. In my dream, I was perfect. I didn't have anything wrong with me. I was no longer in pain. I never saw God, but I heard Him. God said to me, "Mina, you have to go back! You have a destiny you must fulfill!"

And I pleaded with Him, "No, dear God, I don't want to suffer anymore. I'm ready to be with You."

He said, "No, you must go back." In heaven, I was perfect. There are no words for how peaceful it was there. At that very instant, I woke up.

When I came to, all these doctors were around me. People were placing a blood pressure cuff on my arm, giving me oxygen, and putting a pill under my tongue. The doctor asked me, "What happened?"

I said, "Well, when you tell somebody they are going to die, what do you expect to have happen?"

The doctor said, "I didn't tell you were going to die. I told you that if you don't start dialysis, you are going to die."

It may seem a little harsh, but it must be said for my sake and for others: doctors need to have compassion and empathy for those in their care. I know it isn't always easy. Don't get me wrong. I am not asking for sympathy. I am asking that people think before they speak. On the day that my life changed, I didn't need an insensitive, uncaring doctor. What I needed was a compassionate human being who happened to be a doctor.

Not only do I want this book to educate patients, but I also want it to teach doctors to show compassion. These patients, including myself, are full of fear. How doctors speak to a person can make or break their approach to healing.

CHAPTER 4

First and Second Stages of Loss and Grief

In January 1992, I woke up to a new beginning. I woke up to a new life. Once my blood pressure was stabilized, the doctor continued to tell me that I had kidney failure. I was going to start hemodialysis, and they were going to put me on a renal diet. I looked at him with fear in my eyes. I wanted to ask him what that meant. What was hemodialysis? What was a dialysis machine? I could not get the words out. Panic took over my whole being, and I was paralyzed with fear. All I knew was that I was going to die. I remember being afraid of the unknown.

Prior to my illness, my husband had not been there for me. He would not take care of the kids, not even when they had a cold. Now, during the entire time I had been in the hospital, this man was suddenly by my side at all times. The person I thought wasn't going to be there for me was there for me 110 percent. He had to work eight or nine hours a day, come home, and take care of the kids. My husband worked the late shift, would go and get a few hours of sleep, and then spend the rest of the morning with me at the hospital.

I don't know how my husband did it, but he was suddenly my rock. When you are so afraid, you really need someone to be there with you, to hold and just comfort you. You don't need pity; you just need someone to be your rock. He was my best friend, the man I longed for. My prince had finally arrived. I remember he would tell me over and over again, "You know, Mina, God made big crosses for big bosses and then He made little crosses for people named Mina. You have to hang on."

In the beginning of our marriage, he was never there, not even for Christmas. Suddenly, this man stuck by me through my illness. It was a new beginning of my life. It was another chapter.

I had no social worker, no dietician, absolutely no education at all. This was a hospital where they had great specialists and great doctors, yet no one to be the person I needed them to be for me. I remember that a social worker came into my room and said, "Oh my God, you look like a scared little puppy."

With tears streaming down my face, I said, "I'm going to die."

And the social worker asked, "What do you mean you're going to die?"

I said, "They told me that I'm going to start dialysis, and I don't even know what that is." So she sat with me and explained to me what dialysis was. She explained that they are going to put a graft in my arm and then utilize it to put needles in my arm through which they were going to dialyze me. She went on to say that this would take care of only twenty percent of the job of my kidneys because they were no longer working. A very simple explanation, but it didn't quite take the fear away.

Later, they put the dialysis graft in my forearm and sent me home. I had to begin hemodialysis three times a week for three hours at a time. Before I left the hospital, someone had mentioned to me something about a dialysis support group. I called the social worker of that support group, Melissa. I told her I would be at the meetings, and she welcomed me openly. Everyone in the support group was so nice and friendly. They all started showing their arms and scars and telling me it was going to be okay. I was in deep denial. I just smiled and nodded. I remember saying to myself, *"Oh my God, I am not going to be like these people. No, no, no! From now on, I promise to start taking care of my blood pressure! From now on I'm going to take better care of myself, and I will not have to start this thing called dialysis!"*

The social worker at the hospital told me that my kidney function was gone and that I needed the dialysis machine to clean my blood. My kidneys were not able to produce any hormones. I was always tired because I was anemic. My kidneys were not able to perform any of their normal functions. This is why I needed dialysis, but I heard only what I wanted to hear and nothing else. My whole life was turned upside down; it was a tough time for me.

When I first attended my support group, I looked down on the other members. I figured I would take my blood pressure medicine, my kidneys would heal, and I would be all better. I wasn't one of them. I didn't know that once the kidneys stopped working, that was it—there's no going back. I was in deep denial.

I don't remember being angry. I remember being depressed and losing hope. I remember thinking I wanted to be there for my sons' graduations. I remember being in denial, but I don't remember being angry. I had to take care of my mom, my grandson Ritchie, and myself, and I didn't have time to be angry. Now, I speak to my patients about anger all the time.

CHAPTER 5

The Beginning of a New Ending

Nobody can go back and start a new beginning, but everyone can start today to make a new ending.

—Maria Robinson

The first time I went to a dialysis center was in Los Angeles during the Rodney King trial result and the riots. I needed a doctor's permit to go into the city because there was a curfew. There was heavy police presence. I could hear gunshots and fire engines, and smoke was heavy in the air. It was scary enough that I had to put up with the riots, but I also had to start dialysis. I saw patients sitting in chairs: some were reading, others were watching television, and a few were eating lunch. I saw the red tubes and realized it was the blood being recycled. I was afraid and felt like

I was in a nightmare and I was going to wake up at any second. My body was full of toxins, and I was really quite confused, so I don't remember much of the dialysis that went on in Los Angeles. What I do remember, though, is that when they started to put the needles in my arm, I held my breath and nearly passed out.

I was at the center in Los Angeles for a few months before they could transfer me to a facility closer to home. I was finally sent to Glendora, California. At this center was a wonderful nurse named Lily who always had a big smile, a hug, and a kind word. Lily went above and beyond her duty. She would sit and talk or give me a big hug if I needed it. When I was ready to quit, she would come into my room, lighting it up like sunshine itself. She was so kind to me and to all of her patients and their families. I appreciated her kindness and empathy. Lily was a mentor to me, and I have transferred what she taught me to my own clients.

> The greatest pleasure in life is doing what others say you cannot do.
>
> —Walter Baghot

My health was very stable for about a year, so I started adult education classes at a vocational school near our home. I wanted to become a medical assistant. However, that involved a lot of time at school, and the schedule was grueling and required a lot of energy I didn't have. My counselor suggested that I could take some computer classes to brush up on my skills. This is a part of a paper I wrote while I was in school:

What education means to me?

Going back to school has been a wonderful and rewarding experience. Now I have the desire to further my education, and soon I will obtain the skills to do so. Every day, I have a sense of accomplishment. I also have terrific teachers who show me how to do the best and be the best I can be. Education is a privilege that no one should take for granted. One year ago, I found myself in a hospital bed; the doctors announced to me that I had kidney failure. After weeks of depression, I decided to put my life back on track. Now slowly I am gaining my confidence and self-esteem.

As sometimes happens, a monkey wrench was thrown into the mix. Complications started to set in, one after another. I felt like I had been riding a roller coaster for these years, and as soon as I put my foot on the ground, the roller coaster would go for another spin. My graft was no longer working—it was clotted.

I went through this for four years, in and out of the hospital, in and out of the emergency room. I would be dialyzed at the dialysis center for maybe three or four weeks and then the graft would clot again. Back to the hospital I would go. There were no other places on my arms. They had utilized both my forearms and upper arms, so they placed the new graft in my upper thigh. Then they ran out of places on my legs.

I was running out of options. The doctor told me, "You know, Mina, there's a doctor at UCLA who has done five hundred angioplasty procedures. The procedure is simple: he puts in a needle and injects dye through your veins to see what is clotting the vein and if he can clear the clot or blockage. He's a wonderful doctor. He's done this procedure many times, and we have no reason to believe this procedure wouldn't work for you. Your worries will be over."

At Kaiser, they put me in a bed and injected dye through my body. It was supposed to make my dialysis run smoothly. After the procedure was over, I was still in a semiconscious state when the doctor came by my bed and said, "I'm sorry, Mina, but it didn't work." Of five hundred patients who had gone through this procedure and were successful, number 501 was the one who wasn't so lucky. That was me!

Chapter 6

My True Second Chance at Life

At the time, only one friend asked me how I was. We had been friends since junior high. All of my other friends seemed to have disappeared. I wasn't fun to be around anymore. I was always depressed, and I was always crying. Why would anyone want to talk to me? I think it wasn't that they didn't want to talk to me or that they didn't care. It was simply that they were afraid of their own mortality. If it could happen to me, it could happen to them.

I was losing hope. I basically didn't have a life. I wanted to live so badly. I wanted to see my kids grow up, and I wanted to be around when they had kids so I could be a grandma. I knew I was running out of time, and I knew that I wasn't going to live long, so I began to bargain with God.

I recall it was around Thanksgiving that I asked God to please let me live long enough to see my kids graduate from high school. Thanksgiving came and went. The next thing I knew, it was Christmas, and I was back in the hospital. Christmas is extra special to me now, because it seemed I spent every holiday in the hospital. I love Christmas Eve, and I love being with my family. Just one day with absolute peace. No arguing or complaining—just being together as a family. This Christmas, though, I was back in the hospital.

The complications continued, but I got to see both of my sons graduate. I was grateful.

In 1993, when I was on hemodialysis, one of my sons told me that his girlfriend was pregnant. At that time, I said to myself, *"Oh my God, my son has a full scholarship to go to college, and I really want him to attend college. What is he going to do with the baby? He's only seventeen."* I just didn't know what to think or what to do, but God had a plan. You have to follow His kindness, and you have to trust Him. A lot the time, our lives are like a movie: we don't know the end, but God does. I'm very proud of my son. As everyone knows, we make mistakes. It is not shameful to make a mistake and admit that you've made a mistake, but it is shameful to make a mistake and to continue to make it over and over again. The mistakes he made have made him the good man he is today.

When I passed out when the doctors first told me I had kidney failure, I dreamt I spoke to God. He said that I had a destiny to fulfill. This was part of what He meant. My son's girlfriend gave birth to their son, a beautiful little boy with green eyes like his dad's. He was so skinny and had long legs. He was a baby full of life, and there I was losing my life. My grandson came to live with us, and he gave me hope—something to hold on to.

Not only did I get to see my sons graduate, but I also got to see my grandson graduate from high school. He has his driver's license. He has a job, and he is going to attend college and become a pediatrician. When he was five and watching the "Powerpuff Girls," I told him to turn off the television. Defiantly, he told me the Powerpuff Girls were going to save the world. I said, "I'll make a deal with you. I'll put the timer on, and when it goes off, you have to go to sleep." I closed my eyes so he would stop talking to me. He got up, covered me, and gave me a soft kiss on my cheek. He said, "I love you, and thank you, Grandma, for being there for me." I then knew what God meant in my dream. Everything I went through was to learn the lessons that were presented and to take care of that little baby. My grandson needed me, and I was there for him in the midst of my own despair.

I am very proud of all my grandkids. I have three more beautiful grandkids in addition to my eldest grandson, Richard.

Dominique is full of sunshine and love. She is a very caring, very special little girl and never a problem for her mom and dad. Jesse is a mama's boy, and he is a good kid. He's funny and full of life. Anthony is quite handsome and so proud. He is going to be a heartbreaker, and he is very smart.

As my health was declining further, I felt so tired and so sick. One day, I told my husband, "Richard, I am so ready to quit. I don't want to die, God knows I don't want to die, but I don't want to live like this anymore. I'm not alive, and I'm not dead. I'm somewhere in between." After speaking with my husband, we decided to speak to a social worker.

First, though, we talked to my nurse. She said, "Mina, the only thing we can do is put you in the hospital, give you an IV, and then take you completely off dialysis. You will die within three to five days. We will keep you comfortable the entire time."

I then spoke to my friend Melissa, a social worker at the first support group that I had attended. Angrily, she said, "Mina, how selfish of you. I never thought of you as a selfish person. What if you don't die and you become a vegetable? You will only burden your family." At the time, I didn't know she was lying, but she had to say what she said to keep me alive. Later, I told her I knew she had lied. She simply said, "Quit whining, quit complaining, you're alive!"

The nurse offered me a new solution called peritoneal dialysis, which is done at home. A tube is inserted in your peritoneum cavity. A solution is put in your body, and the solution is drained for twelve hours during the night. One exchange (treatment) a day is required. I started peritoneal dialysis, and as soon as the catheter was placed in my peritoneum cavity, I gained my life back. Miracles do exist, but they come in many different forms. It's up to you to keep the miracle alive by being a compliant patient.

During most of my dialysis journey, I kept a journal to help me sort my feelings and to get my thoughts out. Here are several entries.

January 3, 1995, at 6:15 p.m.

Dear God, thank you for one more year of life, I didn't think I was going to make it to see the New Year, but with your help and the help of my family, I made it. There is a lot of fear in my life and a lot of hope. There is a lot of love from my family.

January 14, 1996, at 6:30 p.m.

Well, dear God, I got to see another year. I have been doing peritoneal dialysis today. Dear God, my body is working for me and not against me. Every day, I feel stronger and stronger. Dear God, thank you because I have such a loving and caring family. Today, Carlos vacuumed the whole house, and he made hamburgers for lunch. Every day, I thank God I have a loving and caring family.

I was on peritoneal for two years. I was able to drink more water. Eat beans. (I'm Mexican; I needed to have my beans). I went back to school since I was regaining my strength. I went once a week and then I started twice a week as I gained more strength. I started to volunteer first with the National Kidney Foundation and then with the American Association of Kidney Patients. More complications set in, though: the peritoneal stopped working for me, and my blood pressure was now dropping. I was panicked and scared. It was time to get back on the roller coaster.

CHAPTER 7

From Despair to Hope

On February 19, 1998, without knowing it, my life was going to change again. The morning went on like any other morning. Even though I was stable on peritoneal dialysis, my blood pressure ranged from high to low. That day was a low blood pressure day. I did a few dishes and a little cleaning. By midday, I was already tired. Little Richie, my grandson, had gone to spend the weekend with his parents, so I was basically by myself. My husband was still working nights, so he was asleep.

Beyond the aforementioned chores, my day consisted of watching television and reading. As night approached, I had dinner and went upstairs to take a shower and hook myself to my peritoneal dialysis (continued cycling dialysis). I was watching television and must have fallen asleep. I was awakened by the sound of the phone ringing around ten. It was UCLA calling, saying there was kidney available, a near-perfect match. Not everyone gets a second chance in life. There are more than eighty-nine thousand people currently waiting for a kidney transplant in the United States, and here was a near-perfect match just for me.

I was advised to call my husband immediately and to continue dialysis until further notice. I had paged my husband 911 on his pager. (At that time, we didn't have cell phones.) I called my sons, and they were both at the house within a half hour. My husband immediately came home. I realized that I had been sick with the flu within the last two weeks. Once again, I think God was watching over me because I immediately became very calm and realized that even though they may not be able to go through with the surgery, I was at least at top of the list.

When I got to UCLA around eleven that night UCLA called back and gave the okay to come in to the hospitcal. The elevators were not working, so I had to go up three flights of stairs. Immediately, the doctors began conducting their preliminary testing to ensure that they could move forward with the surgery. Within a very short time, the doctors said they were ready to go and that my body was free of any virus. As the doctors continued their exams, I saw the helicopter land. The medic had a little red ice chest in his hand, and I knew that inside it was my new kidney. I was transferred to the operating room. According to my husband, the surgery lasted between four and six hours. He tells me now that he was very worried about what could happen. When I woke up from surgery, I was in no pain and felt as though I had been born again. I was in intensive care for a few hours and then transferred to a room.

The following day, the social worker came into my room and told me that my donor had been thirteen years old and died as a result of an accidental shooting. My family was happy and full of joy because I had a second chance at life, but somewhere a family was grieving a loved one and planning a funeral. On that day, I promised God and the little boy that his life was not going to be in vain. I was going to educate others regarding organ donation, and to this day, I have kept my promise. The only way to say thank you is to continue my mission—to educate the public in organ donation. Someday, I will have the honor of meeting my organ donor's family. The following poem, a Jewish remembrance, expresses my feelings for them. It sums up my sentiments and what I might say to his family. My hope is they and all those who read it find solace in the words and peace in their hearts and souls. Use it as a prayer and as a motivation to consider becoming a donor. You, too, can be a donor angel. You can share the gift of life. Have a heart, and share a part of yourself.

We Remember Them

In the rising of the sun and in its going down, we remember them.

In the blowing of the wind and the chill of winter, we remember them.

In the warmth of the sun and the peace of summer, we remember them.

In the rustling of the leaves and the beauty of autumn, we remember them.

In the beginning of the year and when it ends, we remember them.

When we are weary and in need of strength, we remember them.

When we are lost and sick at heart, we remember them.

When we have joys we yearn to share, we remember them.

So as long as we live, they too shall live,

For they are now a part of us,

As we remember.

When I first received my transplant, it was a big adjustment for my family. Before my transplant, I was in bed a lot. I was always dependent on someone because I was so sick. I am very grateful to everyone who helped me along the way, especially my family. After the transplant, though, I was like a dog let out of the doggie door. They couldn't keep me in the house. I was doing speaking engagements and traveling. I was always doing something. Sometimes it seemed as though I didn't have enough time to do the things I wanted to do.

Because of this, my husband was feeling left out. After all, he had been my caretaker for the previous seven years. Now that I was always busy, I wasn't thinking that he would have felt that way. It was very hard for him to understand that I wasn't neglecting him, that I did love him, and that I wasn't ungrateful. It was because I was so grateful and so full of joy that I wanted to fulfill my destiny. I was oblivious to the fact that I was hurting the man I loved. We went through a great deal of adjustment. I would be lying if I said I had slowed down—I'm actually doing more. Every time I promote organ donation and someone signs a donor card, I tell my angel, "Okay, we did it! We got someone else to be an organ donor!"

You are stronger than you think—remember to stand tall. Every challenge in your life helps you to grow. Every problem you encounter strengthens your mind and your soul. Every trouble you overcome increases your understanding of life.

—Mina Gonzales

When I felt all was lost, a miracle happened. Life is amazing, and it's what we make of it that counts. We do have choices: we can sit in the corner and feel sorry for ourselves, or we can get up, dust ourselves off, and go forward with life.

Once I received my transplant and regained my strength, I went back to school. I was able to accomplish my goal of becoming a medical assistant. In 2000, I began to volunteer for the American Association of Kidney Patients, serving as vice president. In 2005, I became a Donate Life Ambassador for OneLegacy, an organ—and tissue-recovery organization serving the greater Los Angeles area. Recently, I worked as a peer educator at the Mendez National Institute of Transplantation. I am now mentoring and educating dialysis patients about their options for transplantation. Today, I have the perfect job: I get to sit with patients, thirty minutes at a time, and offer them hope and encouragement. I have an immediate connection with dialysis patients because I was there—I was one of them. I want them to see a miracle in progress. I was a radio host on the web for a show called the Second Chance Show.

In 2010, I was honored to be selected to ride on the Donate Life Rose Parade float. The vote was unanimous. It was such an honor to have been selected, and as a surprise, we met the Rose Parade Queen and her royal court. We also received a tour of the Tournament House.

Once again, my insecurities kicked in. I worried about what would happen if it were a long day or if it rained or that I wouldn't be able handle the hectic day. A shuttle bus was sent for float riders and I, the morning of the parade. We excitedly stepped onto the bus and were whisked away to Vons supermarket. On the way to the market I saw the most glorious sunrise. When we got there, the entire staff was wearing Donate Life shirts, and there was a continental breakfast for us! I knew that the day was going to be fine and that my organ donor was by my side in spirit. I got on the float, and what an honor it was. People were crying and shouting at us, thanking us for bringing organ donation to people's attention and promoting awareness of it. It was beautiful! I saw my transplant coordinator waving at me. It was very emotional. When we got back on the bus after the parade, there was a lot of excitement. We were all talking to reporters on our cell phones about the day's events. I will always treasure remember that day. My angel and I had taken this journey together.

Now, I am a motivational speaker, and my husband and I have traveled across the country. One day, I was in Tampa, Florida, doing a speaking engagement for the American Association of Kidney Patients. Before I spoke, I had to go to the bathroom, and there were about five hundred to seven hundred people waiting for me. When I came out of the bathroom, my dress was tucked in my underwear. As I was about to open the door to the podium, someone yelled at me about my dilemma. Whew! That was a close one!

I received the Mountsatsos Family Comeback Award. It was presented to me for extraordinary courage for overcoming obstacles and providing examples to others. It was presented to me in Tampa by the American Association of Kidney Patients. It was quite a surprise and honor. I was selected out of many deserving volunteers.

On the way home after this conference, there was a thunderstorm, and we had to stop over in Denver. We thought we were going to have to stay the night at the airport, but they gave us vouchers for a hotel and breakfast the next morning. We finally got to Los Angeles, and we found out the airline had lost our luggage. They thought they may have lost it in Denver, but no one was sure. People were yelling and screaming—most of the passengers on our flight had the same dilemma. Watching all this, I was very grateful. I was sitting back and watching all of this commotion, knowing material things can be replaced. On the positive side, we got one more day of vacation. The most important thing, though, I had with me was my angel, my donor. I am quite afraid of flying, but throughout the entire flight, I was calm because I felt his presence. People don't realize that their lives can change in an instant. Minor things like lost luggage are no longer so important.

Breathe as if you were going to live forever, live as if you were going to die today.

—James Dean

How appropriate.

I am living life now, not planning a funeral. Hopefully, I have inspired you to make a good choice. Dialysis can be easy for some. I know plenty who go to work every day and dialyze after work. There are many stories that won't be told because people don't want to scare you. I am only telling you my truth and how I dealt with it. I believe, with certainty, that everything happens for a reason. It's what you do with it that counts. My son tells me that I'm like a bulldog. Once I hold on to something, I don't let it go. Here he writes about how he felt when I was on dialysis and what my transplant means to him:

My mom always cared for me when I was sick as a child with frequent asthma attacks and seizures. When my mom told us about her kidney failure and her need to be on dialysis, I really didn't know what that meant. I felt like I had to return the favor, so for a child of the age of twelve, that meant cleaning the house and making some not-so-yummy eggs for my mom, who ate them anyway because that's the kind of mom she is.

I didn't like seeing my mom suffer the effects of dialysis or worrying whether she would or wouldn't get her kidney transplant. I would wish I could sing her a song or tell her a story to make her feel better, like she used to when I was sick.

When my mom got her transplant, she was so happy and nervous, and I remember feeling the same way. I believe the story of my mom and her transplant begins with all the wonderful work she has done for other people. She has been relentless on educating people and their families on kidney failure and transplantation. She was given the gift of life and did not sit on the sidelines. She went out there and took over the game, and her game plan was educating the uneducated on kidney failure and transplantation and to show people there is life after transplantation.

Richard, my eldest grandson, wrote me a letter explaining how he felt over the course of my illness. I would like to share it with you:

When I lived with my grandma, I remember I would go to school. When I got home, she would get me a snack and then help me with my homework. All I really remember from her being on dialysis is that she would be hooked up to a hospital machine with an IV bag on it. I didn't know if that machine cleaned her blood or what exactly it was used for, but it's amazing that she would be on dialysis and still look after me. I am quite amazed that my grandma has accomplished so much since she got her kidney and has survived what would be a slim chance of survival. She is fifteen years strong, given the fact that most kidneys last between six and eight years, and now she spreads her knowledge of transplantation and gives people hope of new life. I don't know what I would have done without my grandma. She has given me so much in my life, and I love her so much. I'm glad the dialysis machine gave her the time to get her transplant. For my grandma, I will always be her little Richie.

Throughout my entire experience, I was not afraid of dying. I was afraid of living in the uncertainty of what tomorrow would bring. Was it going to be a good dialysis treatment, or was I going to be able to dialyze that day? Was I going to be sent to the emergency room for another procedure to unclot my graft or for emergency surgery? I was afraid of leaving my children. I was afraid of leaving little Richie—he was so small, and he needed me so much. At the same time, though, I was tired of the day-to-day struggle I had to face. What helped me get through those days was my faith in God. He carried me through. Keeping a journal also helped. It helped me to write down my good and bad days. I recommend that all patients do the same. I asked God to help me with the courage to fight for my life for one more day and to give me one more opportunity to see the sunrise and sunset.

I am not defined by my pain, disappointments, or my many setbacks. Today, I define myself by my courage to keep fighting, to see beyond, and to count my many blessings. To quit would have been the easy road. For every problem you encounter and overcome, your understanding of life increases. Remember to stand tall and proud, and go forward. My son Richard wrote the following, and I think it is appropriate to share it here:

When my wife and I got married in the Catholic church, we had to attend a one-day retreat focusing on marriage. When the married couple who was giving the retreat asked us to draw a picture that described our childhood, my picture was a picture of balloons and stick figures laughing. I'm not saying that my life as a kid was all fun and balloons, but rather, that is how my family dealt with fear and uncertainty. The thing that sticks out in my mother's ordeal with kidney failure was how she, and more so my dad, made jokes about the doctors, staff, the dialysis equipment, and more. I know that my mom's ordeal was not a laughing matter, but this is how my parents sheltered us from the pain and uncertainty that my mom was going through. It worked. Today, when I think back on all I the trauma and ordeals my mother faced all alone, I can see how close to the edge we children were to losing our mother and the tremendous sacrifice my mother and father made by withholding their true feelings of fear, uncertainty, and loneliness on our behalf. This is the true strength of my mother, not the fact that she battled doctors and crazed staff, not the fact that she stood up for patient's rights and started various kidney organizations. The greatest achievement that my mother made was protecting her children from the psychological and physical pain that a kidney patient must face.

I have learned so much in life. I have learned I must come first: if I don't take care of myself, I can't take care of others. I have learned that it doesn't matter if someone puts you down. It's not about how they feel about you—it's how they see themselves and their own insecurities. I have learned that you have to learn something new every day. I have learned to appreciate every second of my life. I have learned that you have to follow your dreams, even though other people will put you down for it. Could it be that you are going forward and they are standing still? I have learned to appreciate my family, and I am still in the learning process. Even though I tell them I love them every day, I wonder how many times they really have heard me. I learned to love people who don't know how to love themselves.

I learned was to be my own advocate. I couldn't be shy when I needed something. I had to ask for it. Through all the accomplishments I have had in life, I go back to the scared little girl always looking for her mother's approval. When I go back, I have to remind myself to go forward and leave the past behind. I know now that there is a new beginning every day. I know because I've seen more than fifteen years of new beginnings since my transplant.

Here is the last entry from my private diary;

Today is February 9, 2013 and on February 19, 2013, it will be fifteen years since I had a kidney transplant. I have been blessed in so many ways, and when I feel sad and depressed, all I have to do is count my blessings. I have nothing to complain about. This is a neat little tool, cable, at our house. Richard had been working all night, and he was very tired. So he got upset over the fact that we had to move things around in order for the cable to be installed. There was a lot of yelling. I stayed out of his way and went outside and gave myself a timeout. Just for fifteen minutes. That was enough time for me to look at the sky and look at the people passing by. And then I went inside. By the afternoon, I too lost my temper. I was yelling, too. Don't let anybody control your day. Nobody has the power to ruin your day, control your life, and ruin your destiny, so take a deep breath and just walk away. God has given me so many blessings that I won't allow anyone to ruin my day. I took the easy way out. I didn't need to be right all the time. Let other people be right and keep the peace in your mind and in your heart. Every time I feel like I'm going to lose my temper, please God, remind me to have peace in my heart. Life is too short to get upset over simple things. I have accomplished so many things in the past fourteen years. I have watched my kids grow up; I'm finishing this book. I have a job that I love. I have wonderful friends; we have a home. When things don't go my way, please remind me to have peace in my life. Thank you, dear Lord for the wonderful years.

Appendices

Pictures

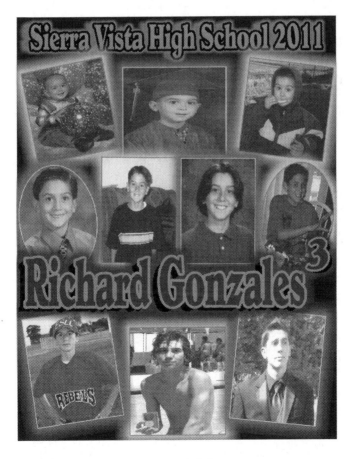

My grandson Richie's life in pictures.

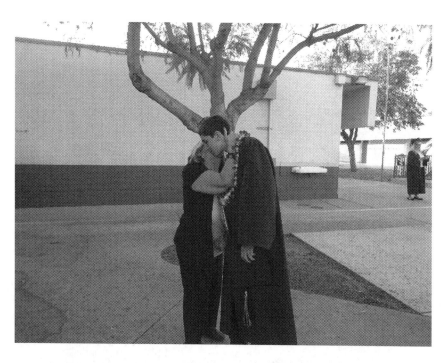

Little Richie's high school graduation from Sierra Vista High.
I am so proud of him.

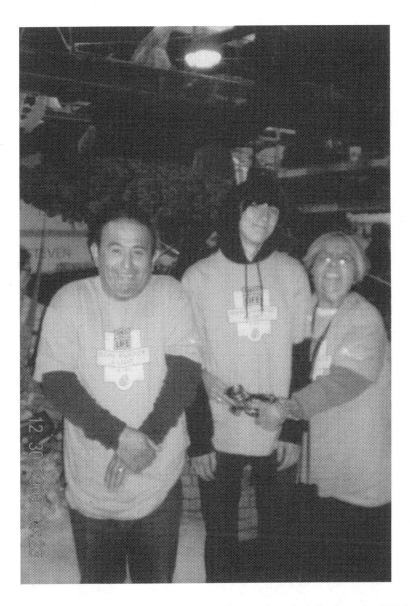

Decorating the OneLegacy Donate Life float a few days before the 2010 Rose Parade. With me are my husband, Richard, and grandson Little Richie.

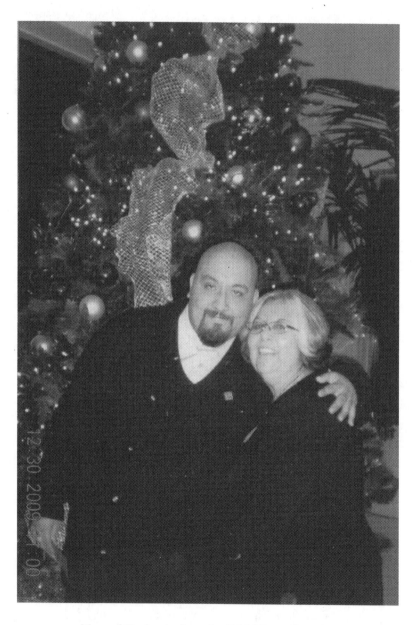

Me and Carlos before the 2010 Rose Parade.

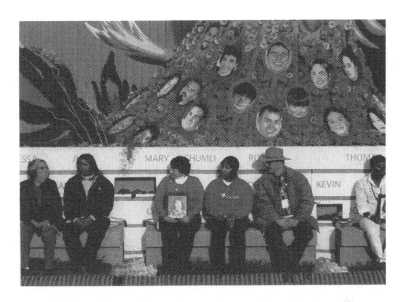

Me and my floatmates at the 2010 Rose Parade riding the OneLegacy Donate Life float. That year's theme was A New Life Rises.

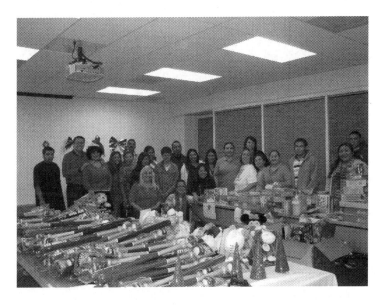

Ambassadors of Donate Life gathering toys to take to the children's hospital for kids on dialysis.

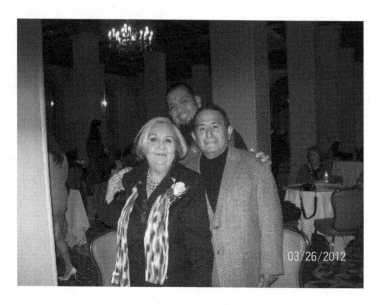

My son Richard, my husband, and me celebrating at the Mujeres
Descatadas dinner and award ceremony.

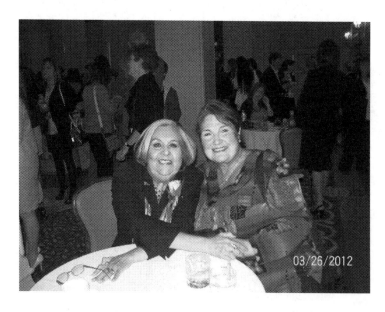

Brenda Chemleski and me at
La Opinion's Mujeres Descatadas award dinner.

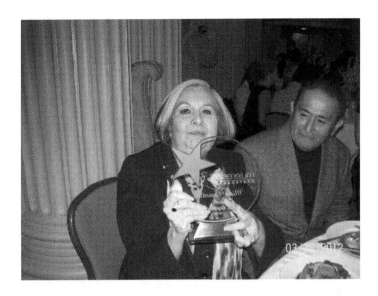

I received the La Opinion's Mujeres Destacadas Award for Educating the Spanish Community on organ donation and organ awareness in 2012.

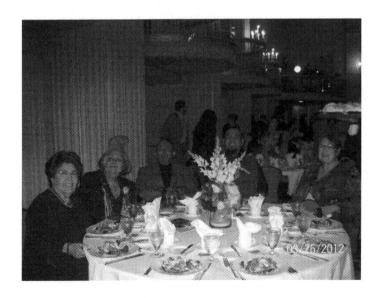

Rachel Rivera, one of my dialysis patients; me; my husband, Richard; my son Richard; and Brenda.

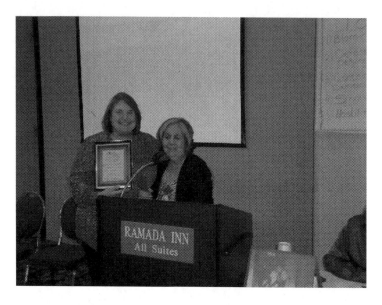

The WIN Global Women's Summit in El Monte, California in 2012.
I am a program director for the WIN, Women's Information Network.

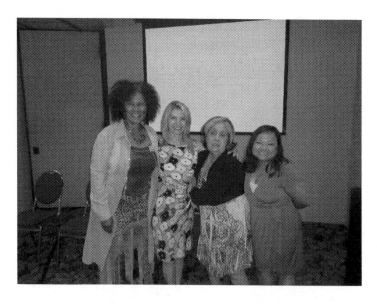

Keynote speaker, Denise L. Cook of the Oracle; Sue Ann Gonis,
Professional Life Coach; me; and my social worker, Jean Bonnette, at the
Global Women's Summit

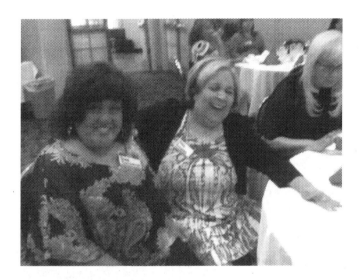

My friend, Dora Calderon at the Global Women's Summit, a platform
I use to educate on kidney health, failure, and transplantation. She
inspires me.

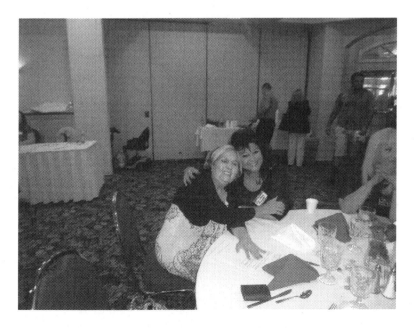

Carolina Meyers and me spending time together at my
Global Women's Summit in 2012.

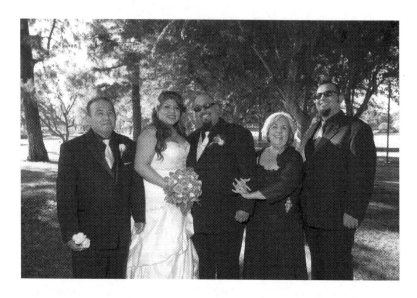

Our family at my son Carlos' wedding.

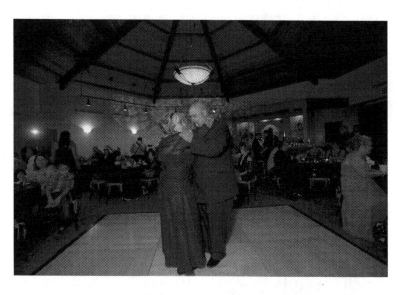

Dancing with my son Carlos on his wedding day. I am happy to be alive.

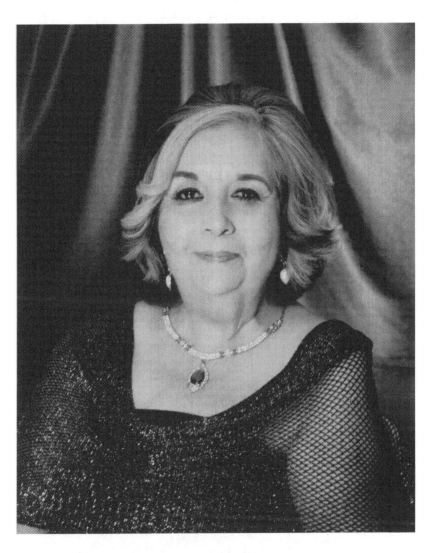
Mina Gonzales
Author, motivational speaker, wife, mother, grandmother, and
kidney transplant survivor.

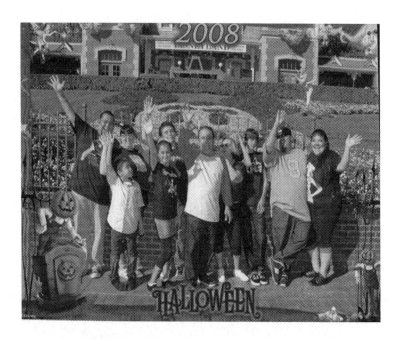

My whole family having a good time at Disneyland.

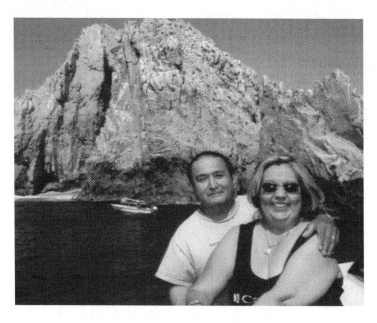

My husband and me on my birthday on a cruise.

GLOSSARY

anemia: A condition that develops when your blood lacks enough healthy red blood cells. These cells are the main transporters of oxygen to organs. If red blood cells are also deficient in hemoglobin, your body isn't getting enough oxygen. Symptoms of anemia such as fatigue occur because organs aren't getting enough oxygen. Anemia is the most common blood condition in the United States. It affects about 3.5 million Americans. Women and people with chronic diseases are at increased risk of anemia.

clotted: Changed from a liquid to a thickened or solid state; coagulated blood.

dialysis machine: The patient's blood is pumped through the blood compartment of a dialyzer, exposing it to a partially permeable membrane. The dialyzer is composed of thousands of tiny synthetic hollow fibers. The fiber wall acts as the semipermeable membrane. Blood flows through the fibers, dialysis solution flows around the outside of the fibers, and water and waste move between these two solutions. The cleansed blood is then returned via a circuit back to the body. Ultrafiltration occurs by increasing the hydrostatic pressure across the dialyzer membrane. This usually is done by applying negative pressure to the dialysate compartment of the dialyzer. This pressure gradient causes water and dissolved solutes to move from blood to dialysate and allows the removal of several liters of excess fluid during a typical three-to five-hour treatment.

graft: A tube that is placed under the skin that attaches one end of the artery to your arm or leg and the other to a vein.

hemodialysis: The process of artificially cleaning waste from the blood. This job is normally done by the kidneys. If the kidneys fail, the blood must be cleaned artificially with special equipment.

kidney: A glandular organ that excretes urea and other waste products; a urinary gland.

kidney failure: Inability of the kidneys to excrete waste and help maintain electrolyte balance.

peritoneal dialysis: The smooth serous membrane that lines the cavity of the abdomen, or the whole body cavity when there is no diaphragm, and, turning back, surrounds the viscera, forming a closed, or nearly closed, sac. The dialysate is transferred into the peritoneal via IV bags. This is performed daily.

renal diet: Consists of a no salt to ensure no fluid retention and maintenance of blood pressure, no phosphorus to ensure healthy bones and heart, limited fluid to ensure heart health and maintain blood pressure, and low potassium for heart health.

transplant: There are two types of donors. For a living-donor kidney transplant, the recipient's diseased or damaged kidneys are usually left in place. The donor's kidney is placed in the recipient's lower abdomen and connected to blood vessels and bladder. The recipient's and donor's surgeries are carried out at the same time in different operating rooms. A cadaver donor is someone who has recently died. Most donor kidneys come from this source. In both cases, the key to success is having the closest possible blood and tissue matches. A family member is not always the best match.

Resources

Axelrod, J. "The Five Stages of Loss and Grief." Psych Central. 2002. http://psychcentral.com/lib/the-5-stages-of-loss-and-grief/000617

Sheps, Sheldon G. *Signs and Symptoms.* Mayo Clinic on High Blood Pressure. Kensington, New York: Mayo Clinic Research, 2002.

Healthwise Staff, Primary Medical Reviewer: Poinier, Anne C, M.D., Internal Medicine. Print.

For more information on organ donation, go to www.donatelife.org or www.unos.org. Also visit www.onelegacy.org, www.donateLIFEcalifornia.org and donevidacalifornia.org.

The following are also helpful sites:

RSN Renal Support Network (www.rsnhope.org)

TRIO Transplant Recipient International Organization (www.trioweb.org)

Needy Meds, (www.needymeds.com)

WebMD (http://www.webmd.com)

UNOS Organ Procurement and Transplant Network optn. transplant.hrsa.gov

ABOUT THE AUTHOR

Mina Gonzales has been a Donate Life Ambassador since 2006, tirelessly representing California's organ and tissue donor registry and educating the public about the donation process and its benefits. As a volunteer, Mina possesses a wonderful combination of both gratitude and action, which motivates her to take the donation message wherever she goes. She generously shares her story in the media, both in English and Spanish, in hospitals, health fairs and any forum where she is invited. After her transplant, Mina made a promise to her donor to honor his gift and his memory, and she has been effectively and faithfully doing that for many years. It is people like Mina who inspire our communities to give the gift of life.

At age forty, Mina Gonzales was enjoying her family life just as any wife and mother would. While attending ballgames with her husband and two young boys, she never dreamed that she was suffering from a silent killer: hypertension.

In January 1992, Mina was admitted to the hospital with extremely high blood pressure. Initially, she was told that she would be there for three days. But those three days turned into a three-month stay as complications arose, including kidney damage. She began dialysis shortly after she was released and was stable for two years.

During the next four years, Mina suffered with every medical complication imaginable and went through every form of treatment. She was placed on the kidney transplant waiting list. Her hope began to fade away, not knowing if she would survive another day. In February 1998, expecting to die before a kidney could be found; Mina received the most important phone call of her life from UCLA Medical Center. They told her they had a perfect match. Thanks to the generosity of her donor's grieving family, despite their loss, her life began again. It was on that day that Mina promised her donor that his life was not going to be in vain. From that day until the present, Mina has kept her promise to dedicate her life to educating others about the importance of organ donation.

In 2000, Mina began volunteering with the American Association of Kidney Patients, serving as vice president. In 2005, she became a volunteer Donate Life Ambassador for One

Legacy, the organ and tissue recovery organization serving the greater Los Angeles area. Currently, she works as a Peer Educator and Motivational Speaker. She feels strongly that the love and appreciation that she has for what was given to her is passed through her volunteering and current employment. Miracles do exist but will come in many different ways. It's up to you to keep the miracle alive by being a compliant patient.